Understanding

ARTHRITIS
& RHEUMATISM

Professor Verna Wright

Published by Family Doctor Publications Limited
in association with the British Medical Association

IMPORTANT NOTICE

This book is intended not as a substitute for personal medical advice but as a supplement to that advice for the patient who wishes to understand more about his or her condition.

Before taking any form of treatment YOU SHOULD ALWAYS CONSULT YOUR MEDICAL PRACTITIONER.

In particular (without limit) you should note that advances in medical science occur rapidly and some of the information about drugs and treatment contained in this booklet may very soon be out of date.

© Family Doctor Publications 1993, 1995
Reprinted 1994
Second edition 1995
Reprinted 2000

Family Doctor Publications, 10 Butchers Row, Banbury, Oxon OX16 8JH

Medical Editor: Dr Tony Smith
Consultant Editor: Chris McLaughlin
Cover Artist: Dave Eastbury
Medical Artist: Angela Christie
Design: Fox Design, Godalming, Surrey
Printing: Reflex Litho, Thetford, using acid-free paper

ISBN: 1 898205 55 8

Contents

Introduction

NO NEED TO GRIN AND BEAR IT

At the age of 52, Mrs Jones, who had never been ill before, developed a nagging pain in her knee. Her friends told her unsympathetically: 'It is just a touch of rheumatism; there's nothing you can do about it so you had better grin and bear it. What do you expect anyway at your age?'

Mrs Jones, however, was one of the 20 million people in the UK who each year suffer from some rheumatic complaint: one in four of all medical consultations at hospitals are for rheumatic diseases, and more than eight million patients consult their family doctors about this.

Fortunately, Mrs Jones's fears were unjustified and her friends' responses were wrong. There was something that she and her doctor could do about the painful knee and she certainly was not going to be crippled.

This booklet aims to give greater knowledge and understanding of rheumatism and arthritis. It endeavours to allay many of the worries that sufferers have and reassure them that modern treatments can be most effective.

Diagnosis

A problem of definition

Although the terms 'rheumatism' and 'arthritis' are widely used by both doctors and patients and we all have a general understanding of the sort of problems to which they refer, they have no precise medical meaning.

Rheumatism is an umbrella term which includes a whole spectrum of disorders (some 200) many of which result in aching muscles and ligaments but do not affect the joints.

Arthritis, on the other hand, is inflammation of one or several joints.

Just to confuse the issue further, however, in the most common form of arthritis – osteoarthritis – there may be little inflammation.

Space does not permit a full list of all the rheumatic or arthritic disorders, but the most common and important of these are dealt with in the next few pages.

Osteoarthritis (osteoarthrosis)

Osteoarthritis normally occurs in older people as a result of wear and tear on joint surfaces, particularly the larger weightbearing joints such as hips, knees or spine. The end joints of fingers, however, are also frequently involved and some people have bunions affected by osteoarthritis on the big toes. More women than men suffer from osteoarthritis and the condition often starts after the menopause.

What happens is that where the smooth lining of the bones come into contact (this is known as articular cartilage) it begins to flake and crack through over-use or, perhaps, injury. As the cartilage deteriorates it affects the bone which can become thickened or distorted. Movement of the joint than becomes painful and restricted and the muscles that move the joint gradually start to waste away.

There may be episodes of pain,

stiffness, and swelling in the affected joint over months or even years. In a few patients the pain becomes severe, but eventually the joint deteriorates and as it becomes stiff it may also become less painful. The extent of swelling in the affected joint varies – in some cases it is scarcely noticeable and in others the joint becomes extremely knobbly. Pain may also be caused by inflammation from minor sprains of the unstable joint or by crystals that are deposited in the joint lining.

The doctor can prescribe drugs which help with pain and inflammation and it is important that patients should take adequate exercise and keep their weight down, thereby taking some of the strain off the joints.

Spondylosis: slipped disc

The spinal column (backbone) stretches from the base of the skull to the bottom of the buttocks and consists of more than 30 separate bones called vertebrae, which are linked by strong ligaments and have flexible discs lying between them. The discs have a strong outer covering around a jellylike inner layer. The spinal cord runs through a channel made up of the vertebrae, and peripheral nerves from this pass through side channels to and from other parts of the body.

Because of its complex structure the spine is very susceptible to mechanical problems such as *spondylosis* or *prolapsed (slipped) disc*. In the former condition some of the spaces between the vertebrae become narrower because the discs have degenerated (through age, over-use, or injury) and lost their elasticity. The spinal column stiffens and loses its flexibility and sometimes bony outgrowths develop on the vertebrae or along the edge of the degenerating discs which may press on various nerves causing pain. If a disc begins to degenerate because of age or back strain, pressure may cause some of the softer centre to squeeze out through a weak point in the fibrous outer layer and result in a loss of the cushioning effect of the disc and painful pressure on a nerve from the squeezed out portion. This is known as a prolapsed or slipped disc.

At other times the combination of osteoarthritis of the small joints between the vertebrae or strained ligaments produces the back pain.

CASE HISTORY

It was a delightful Spring morning when Andrew Jones (aged 25) began to dig his garden. As he turned the third spadeful of earth he was struck by a severe pain in his lower back. He could barely straighten up. Even when he got into the house the pain persisted, and the only comfortable position was lying on the floor. The pain by

What happens to a joint with osteoarthritis?

Normal joint

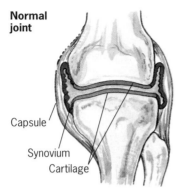

Capsule

Synovium

Cartilage

Early stage

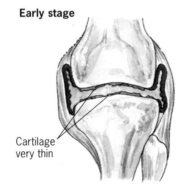

Cartilage very thin

Late stage showing cartilage starting to deteriorate

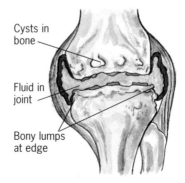

Cysts in bone

Fluid in joint

Bony lumps at edge

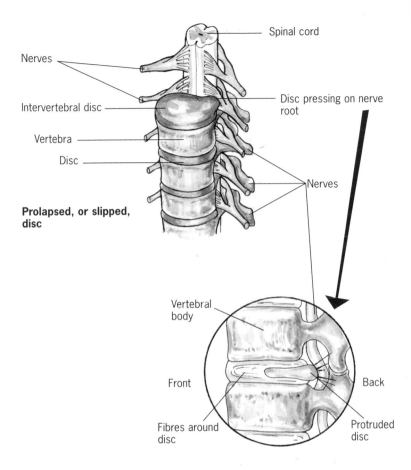

Prolapsed, or slipped, disc

this time was travelling down the back of his leg, and so his wife called his GP. The GP diagnosed a slipped disc with sciatica, advised rest and prescribed a pain-relieving medicine. Andrew had to take two weeks off work, but by the end of this time felt much better. By the end of the third week the pain had gone completely.

Non-specific backache
Not all back pains are mechanical in origin, however, the majority have no obvious cause. Most are probably

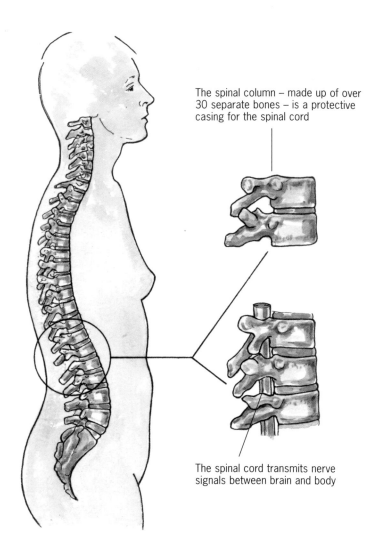

The spinal column – made up of over 30 separate bones – is a protective casing for the spinal cord

The spinal cord transmits nerve signals between brain and body

due to a strained ligament or vertebrae joint that cause surrounding muscles to go into painful spasm, or to fibromyalgia (stiffness and pain felt deep within the muscles caused by any number of factors such as physical strain or emotional tension).

In many cases the best course is to take a painkiller such as paracetamol. Take these regularly every four hours during the day (but not more than eight in 24 hours) to help control the pain. Apply heat with a hot water bottle wrapped in cloth, and rest on a bed with a hard mattress – or put some boards or plywood under the mattress. Do not become discouraged; give the painkillers time to work. If the backache persists for more than three days you should consult a doctor.

NON-ARTICULAR RHEUMATISM

As the name suggests, conditions grouped under this heading are not arthritis. They include:

Tennis/golfer's elbow

Tennis elbow is the term used to describe damage to the muscle tendon in the elbow where it joins the upper arm bone (humerus), causing pain on the outer side of the elbow. If the pain is on the inner side of the elbow the condition is called golfer's elbow. Usually there is an obvious link with over-use of the muscles, though not necessarily at tennis or golf. It could be a knitting machine, for example.

CASE HISTORY

Mrs Pauline Nevin was looking forward to her holiday as she carried a particularly heavy suitcase along the railway platform. As she did so, she began to feel the outside of her elbow become increasingly painful. It got so bad that she had to buy a luggage trolley to carry her case to the taxi, and she wished she had bought one earlier. What Mrs Nevin was experiencing was a tennis elbow. Her elbow continued to be painful for several weeks after that, although it gradually improved. Even now, however, she still gets the pain sometimes when she carries anything heavy.

Frozen shoulder

People in their 40s commonly suffer from a painful condition sometimes called periarthritis of the shoulder or frozen shoulder (so called because the normal range of movement is impossible because of this condition).

Inflammation around it produces pain and an inability to move the arm above the head or behind the back leading to disuse, which in turn causes more stiffness and pain.

Sometimes an injury brings it on or it may be caused by repetitive movements or unaccustomed exer-

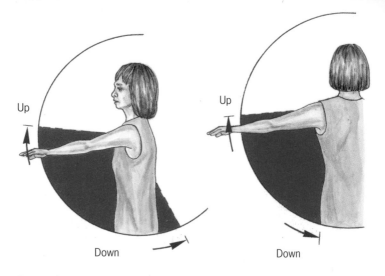

Up

Down

Up

Down

Range of movement may be restricted because of a frozen shoulder

cise. Often the condition seems to come out of the blue. It is important to seek professional help for a frozen shoulder because mobility may be permanently impaired if it is left untreated for too long.

Another common shoulder disorder at this age is a rotator cuff lesion. When this happens part of the muscle complex around the shoulder becomes damaged. Some of the shoulder movements are painful, particularly if they are resisted.

Housemaid's knee

You don't have to be a housemaid to experience this problem! In fact coal miners were commonly affected, when the condition was called bear knee.

Joints often have a small sac containing a little fluid (a bursa) adjacent to them to ease movement of tendons or skin over a bony prominence. If the bursa is irritated by pressure or by injury it may become inflamed and fill with excess fluid (bursitis). The most common example of this is housemaid's knee, in which the bursa in front of the knee-cap (patella) swells and becomes painful. Other joints particularly susceptible to this disorder include the elbows, heels, base of the big toe and the shoulders. Bursitis is not a serious disorder and if pressure is kept off the joint it should clear up within a week or so. If it persists, consult your doctor.

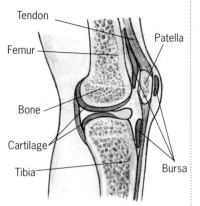

Knee joint showing signs of bursitis, or housemaid's knee

Muscular pains

Some pains may be muscular in origin. Muscle tension, often caused by anxiety or overwork, sometimes produces pain around the neck and shoulder girdle and poor posture may also be a contributory factor. Some of these conditions have been called fibrositis or fibromyalgia, medical terms for stiffness and pain felt deep within the muscles. This type of pain usually clears up within three or four days and it may be eased by hot baths and painkillers taken regularly for a few days. Sometimes an ice-pack helps.

CASE HISTORY

Clare Williams, a 35-year-old mother of two, found her muscle pains didn't go away. She felt them not only around the neck and shoulder girdle, but down the spine, at the side of the hips and even around the knee. There was nothing to see, but when her doctor pressed on these areas they were tender. Her sleep was disturbed and she didn't feel refreshed when she woke in the morning. She felt generally exhausted and quite disabled. Previously she had suffered from an irritable bowel, which the doctor explained was often associated with this condition – known as fibromyalgia. Her doctor prescribed a small dose of a medication to ease the pain at night. He also explained that she could help herself by following the planned course of exercises he was recommending. Clare stuck to the programme, and fortunately the symptoms steadily cleared up as a result.

Growing pains

In teenage girls especially, rapid remodelling of bones, particularly those in the legs, may cause pain, often known as growing pains. Reassurance that there is nothing wrong should be backed up by a painkiller such as paracetamol to help relieve the pain.

RHEUMATOID ARTHRITIS

Rheumatoid arthritis is a long-term disease of the joints. Inflammation of the lining of the joint (synovium) may progress to joint damage and in a few cases may actually produce deformity.

It is commonly considered a young person's disease, but although a quarter of cases start before the age of 30, the peak age of onset is between 40 and 50. Women are affected three times more often than men.

The joints usually affected are the small ones in the hands and feet (chiefly the knuckle and toe joints) but rheumatoid arthritis can also affect wrists, knees, ankles and neck; both sides of the body are equally involved. It is less common in the spine or hips, which are affected more usually by osteoarthritis.

The disease may begin without symptoms of joint trouble. The sufferer may simply feel off-colour and without appetite and have vague muscular pain. Only later does the pain and swelling start in the joints. In other cases symptoms of joint problems occur suddenly. Whatever the type of onset, sooner or later the joints affected will become swollen, painful and stiff. Characteristically, the joints are particularly stiff and

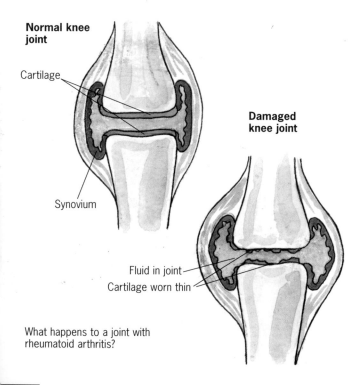

Normal knee joint

Cartilage

Synovium

Damaged knee joint

Fluid in joint

Cartilage worn thin

What happens to a joint with rheumatoid arthritis?

painful first thing in the morning, but these problems ease with exercise as the day goes on. Very occasionally the disease is not limited to the joints; inflammation may also affect the lungs, eyes, and other organs with symptoms such as pleurisy or gritty eyes.

Rheumatoid arthritis is extremely variable in respect of severity, duration and outlook but in actual fact only one sufferer in 10 is severely disabled by the disease and modern treatment can help enormously.

POLYARTHRITIS

Polyarthritis is a term used for any inflammatory condition of several or many joints. The best known is rheumatoid arthritis but there are many other types such as ankylosing spondylitis. Some are associated with a skin condition called psoriasis, some with certain types of colitis, and others, such as the variety that occurs with German measles, last only a few days.

Ankylosing spondylitis

Spondylitis is inflammation of the joints linking the vertebrae. In ankylosing spondylitis the inflammation recedes but results in hardened, damaged joints that effectively fuse the vertebrae together causing pain and restricted back movement in all directions. There is also reduced chest expansion because the rib joints are inflamed where they join the spinal column. The condition usually affects young men; and it often starts with a low backache and stiffness, which are usually at their worst first thing in the morning. In contrast to the patient with a disc problem, the pain is usually worse at rest.

Some people have vague chest pains and, oddly, tenderness under their heels. The eyes may become red and painful. Early diagnosis and treatment are most important for those affected in order to prevent any type of deformity.

CASE HISTORY

During his teens Brian Gavin had suffered from occasional backache. He was a rugby player and considered himself pretty fit, so he put the pains down to lumbago. However, when he was twenty-one the back pain worsened. He felt tight pains round his chest, and coughing and sneezing made them worse. He also felt his spine becoming stiff. These symptoms were worse first thing in the morning, and improved as the day went on and he became more mobile. At the same time his right eye became red and painful. Brian went to see his doctor, who sent him to have an X-ray of the bottom of his back - the sacro-iliac joints. The X-ray confirmed that Brian was suffering from ankylosing spondylitis. The non-steroidal anti-inflammatory drug he was prescribed and the exercise programme he was shown by the physiotherapist made a great difference to the symptoms. Fortunately the eye inflammation settled down on its own after a few days. If it had not improved Brian would have needed to see an ophthalmologist for an expert opinion.

Gout

Gout is the disease beloved by cartoonists but agonising for those who live with it. It caused Sydney Smith, the great wit, to exclaim: 'I feel as if I am walking on my eyeballs'. Gout is one of the most common forms of joint disease: it affects men mostly, usually after puberty, and women mainly after the menopause.

In gout, crystals of uric acid are deposited, the surrounding tissue becomes inflamed, and the inflammation irritates the nerve endings associated with the joint causing extreme pain.

The big toe is classically affected, becoming red, hot, agonisingly painful, and acutely tender (so much so that the sufferer cannot bear the weight of bedclothes on his foot).

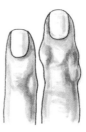

Other joints, such as the fingers, can also be affected by gout.

In subsequent attacks (which not all patients have) other joints may be affected. Sufferers should consult their doctor and should take aspirin as a painkiller. Gout can be controlled very successfully by drugs.

COLLAGEN DISEASES

Connective tissue is an essential part of every structure in the body. The main component of this tissue is collagen. In collagen diseases, which are rare, damage to the collagen in certain areas causes inflammation in which skin, heart, lung, and kidney involvement are more important than the relatively minor associated joint problems. Examples of collagen diseases are systemic sclerosis, systemic lupus erythematosus and polyarteritis nodosa.

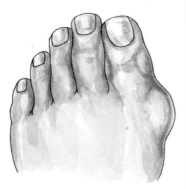

People with these conditions can get more information about them from booklets produced by the Arthritis and Rheumatism Council whose address can be found on page 53.

Polymyalgia rheumatica

This is an important collagen disease recognised in the UK in recent years. It produces considerable stiffness in the shoulder girdles of elderly patients, especially in the mornings. Treatment is dramatically effective.

Why it happens

We do not know the cause of most rheumatic diseases but here are some factors that may predispose to them or make symptoms worse.

Infection

In some cases arthritis may be caused by infection. Arthritis of a single joint can in some cases raise a suspicion of tuberculosis. It may be a reaction to infection such as a sore throat caused by bacteria called streptococci. The latter can produce rheumatic fever three weeks after the throat infection, but fortunately it is not so true any more in Britain today, largely due to public health measures such as better sanitation and less overcrowding.

A few people who have dysentery will develop a reactive arthritis, and this may occur in travellers returning from abroad. Some viral infections such as German measles produce an arthritis just like rheumatoid arthritis but this is short-lived and clears up completely after some weeks.

Excess uric acid

The only arthritis known to be due to excess acid is gout. Too much uric acid in the blood crystallises around the joint and is also deposited elsewhere. These deposits are known as tophi. The false claims that other types of arthritis are caused by acid may needlessly deprive patients of citrus fruits.

Injury

Injury may subsequently produce

AGE

A number of arthritic disorders are caused by wear and tear of joints, but fortunately the change from the supple sapling of 19 to the gnarled oak of 70 is very gradual and only occasionally severely painful.

arthritis in a joint (especially if a fracture goes through the joint itself); it may provoke a flare-up of existing arthritis; or it may cause a general arthritis to localise in a previously damaged joint. An interesting example of the influence of repeated minor trauma was seen in Yorkshire seamstresses who, if they developed generalised osteoarthritis with bony swellings over the end joints of the fingers, were found to have much larger lumps on the right index finger.

Family factors

The likelihood of the children of those who suffer from rheumatic disease being affected is small in most cases.

The risk is somewhat increased with gout, ankylosing spondylitis and arthritis associated with psoriasis and is also rather greater with generalised osteoarthritis. With rheumatoid arthritis the risk is not much more than that for the general population, remembering that this is a common disease and one in every 20 members in a family is likely to develop it by chance (if they live long enough).

Pregnancy

Low back pain often occurs in pregnancy due to laxness of the ligaments and to the altered mechanics of the spine, but this seldom results in long-term problems.

Babies are not in jeopardy by being born to arthritic mothers except for a slightly increased risk of the condition known as systemic lupus erythematosus.

It is generally best to take as few drugs as possible during pregnancy and fortunately most rheumatic diseases go into remission during this time so that drug control is not a problem. The disease often recurs six to twelve weeks after delivery but is no worse than previously.

Try to see your physiotherapist and occupational therapist regularly before you have the baby. They will help you develop ways of coping once the baby is born.

THE WEATHER

Cold and damp weather may make you feel your aches and pains more but does not cause arthritis.

A survey in the West Indies showed that Jamaicans had just as much arthritis as Britons, but complained less. This could have been because the absence of a National Health Service in Jamaica gave little point in complaining, but was more likely due to the warmer climate. Rheumatic sufferers should avoid cold draughts, keep their house warm and dress up warmly in winter.

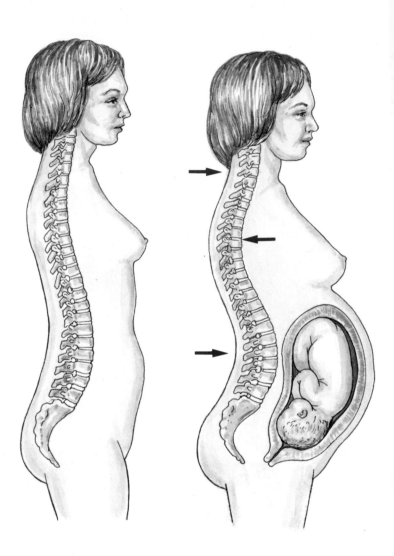

Note how curvature of the spine is different in pregnancy (shown on the right) from normal (on the left)

Investigations

The diagnosis for most rheumatic patients is made by the doctor listening carefully to the symptoms and examining the joints. Other investigations only help to clarify the picture in the more difficult cases or to monitor the course of a disease or the effects of treatment.

Blood tests

Blood tests may be needed to establish the diagnosis; for instance most patients with rheumatoid arthritis have a substance called rheumatoid factor in their blood which can be found on testing. It is worth stressing, however, that five per cent of normal people have this, so its presence does not necessarily confirm the diagnosis.

Gouty patients have a raised blood uric acid concentration. An increased erythrocyte sedimentation rate or plasma viscosity indicate inflammation and the higher the reading, the more active the disease is likely to be.

These tests may also be used to monitor the effects of treatment.

The concentration of uric acid in the blood, for instance, indicates the effect of long-term treatment of gout.

Other tests may show complications of the arthritis or its treatment: a low haemoglobin concentration indicates anaemia; a raised white blood cell count may be due to infection; and a low white blood cell or platelet count may alert the doctor to the side-effects of drug treatment.

They are the most useful diagnostic tests for rheumatoid arthritis and if taken at regular intervals help the doctors or specialist involved to monitor progress of the disease.

Radiography

X-rays may help in diagnosis by showing the state of the joint surface: whether the bone is damaged or whether there are bony outgrowths from the edges of the joint or in the ligaments.

Treatments

Exercises

Exercises are vital for the well-being of arthritic sufferers as they mobilise joints and strengthen muscles and some basic mobility exercises are illustrated in the following pages.

A physiotherapist will show you the proper regimen to follow at home. The best results are obtained if you keep a diary card (for instance, of the exercises done and the amount of weight lifted by the leg), and the physiotherapist checks periodically on your progress.

Activity is not the same as exercise. Many patients think that because they are active at home or at work they need not carry out a specific regimen but this is not the case.

Some exercises such as those for the neck, shoulder girdle and spine are postural; some are designed to mobilise specific joints such as the exercises of the arms and the shoulders; and some strengthen important muscles. A few of the exercises benefit the patient indirectly, such as the tummy muscle strengthening exercises for sufferers from low back pain.

DON'T IGNORE PAIN

As a general rule, do not 'bash through pain regardless'.

Pain is not wholly evil; it is often nature's warning signal to cut back on that activity. If pain persists for more than an hour after an exercise or activity you have done too much; so do less next time.

Similarly, any activity that causes rapid swelling of affected joints is probably excessive (see page 43).

Heat treatment and ice packs

Heat and painkillers before exercise sometimes help you to do them better as warmth relieves pain and

Over pages 20–24, there are illustrations of some exercises that are useful for the arthritis sufferer. These exercises should not be performed if they cause a lot of pain

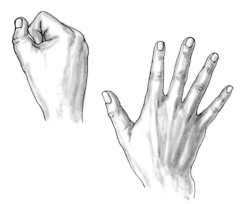

Curl your hand into a fist, squeeze tightly and count to five. Then stretch out your hand and fingers and again count to five. Repeat at intervals throughout the day

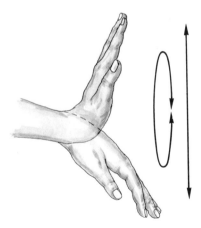

With your arm in a horizontal position, relax your hand so that the wrist is hanging loosely, and then circle your hand first clockwise and then anti-clockwise, so rotating your wrist. Repeat with the other hand

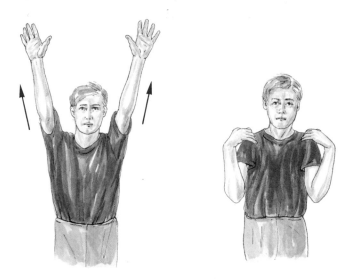

In a standing, sitting or lying position, stretch your arms above your head as far a possible, while breathing in. Hold the position to the count of five. Then breathe out as you lower your arms, bringing your elbows into your body. Repeat these two movements four times in all

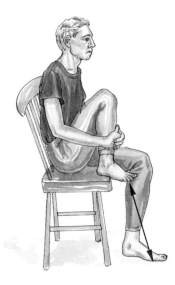

Sitting on a chair, sit straight up and draw up one knee as close as possible to the chest; lower this leg and repeat with the other leg

In a sitting or standing position, drop your chin towards your chest, hold for a count of ten while breathing slowly, and then move your head slowly backwards

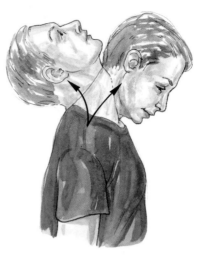

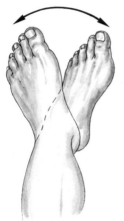

In a sitting position, twist each foot from side to side and then circle slowly clockwise and anti-clockwise

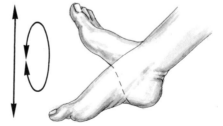

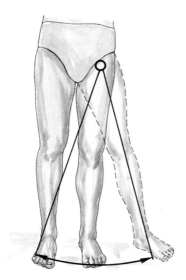

Hip movements outwards and inwards, forwards and backwards. These exercises can be carried out by standing next to a table with the straight leg next to the side. Then stretch the other leg, backwards, forwards and to the side. Repeat this movement four times. Turn and repeat whole sequence with the other leg. This exercise can be carried out in a swimming pool

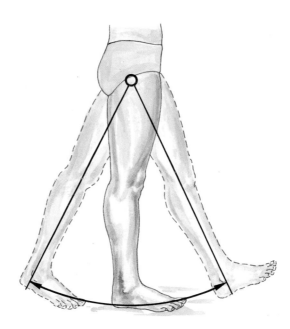

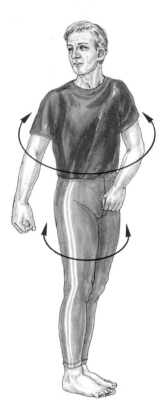

In a standing position, turn your ribs, shoulders and head until you can look behind you or as far round as you can. Hold yourself in this position and count to five. Repeat once in this direction and then twice on the other side

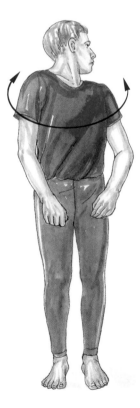

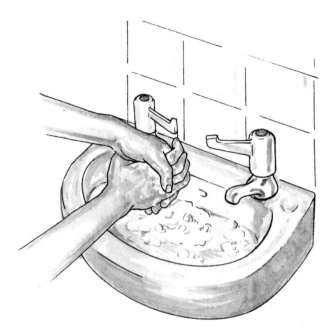

relaxes muscle spasm. Patients with rheumatoid arthritis in the hands should exercise them in hot soapy water first thing in the morning and at other times during the day. A hot

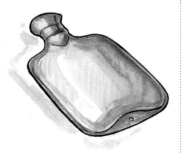

water bottle or cold compress over a painful area may be soothing. A radiant heat lamp can alleviate shoulder girdle pain, but before you buy this expensive equipment borrow one from a friend to see if the treatment suits you. Rheumatic sufferers should take frequent hot baths if they are able. They will find these soothing as they help relax tense muscles and relieve the pain in joints. A shower will also help.

Surprisingly, some people get more relief from ice packs than from heat. A painful frozen shoulder may benefit in this way. A packet of

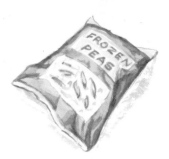

frozen peas taken from the freezer and wrapped in a towel is an easy and extremely practical way of doing this.

Rehabilitation in hospital

Sometimes treatment in hospital is required. The use of hydrotherapy (movements in water, particularly in a deep pool) and other specialist rehabilitation skills often give excellent results. Specialist centres include in their programmes classes for ankylosing spondylitis sufferers for up to a dozen patients at a time. They maintain and increase the mobility of this group of young people. Ideally the patients come in for two or three weeks each year. This one rheumatic disease is above

all others where it is vital to maintain mobility. Spinal and breathing exercises benefit the patient enormously. In the old days they were put in plaster casts in the hope of stopping their spines bending. Inexorably, the spine bent, the cast cracked, and the patient finished with a fixed spinal deformity, often being able to see only the floor. The treatment was entirely wrong for most. Only if a fracture develops in the spine should a cast be used in a patient with ankylosing spondylitis.

Manipulation

The movements discussed above are active: those imposed on a joint by someone else are termed 'passive' and may be achieved by manipulation. In some cases, particularly in the back, dramatic relief may be obtained, but this is relatively rare, and passive movement must always be done carefully and skilfully.

Support

Acute, low back pain (lumbago) must be treated by rest in bed on a firm mattress, preferably with a

REST

During a general flare up of rheumatoid arthritis bed rest may be necessary. During this period all joints should be put through their range of motion daily to prevent them stiffening. Any acutely painful joint needs resting. A painful shoulder may require the arm to be in a sling and a splint may help a painful knee or wrist.

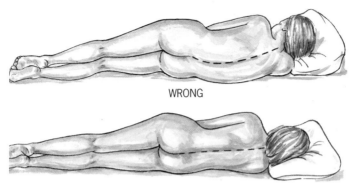

WRONG

RIGHT

board underneath. In severe cases traction (gentle stretching by mechanical means) may be applied to the legs or pelvis. This is a sophisticated and effective way of ensuring rest. A back support or corset helps many long-standing back sufferers and a collar may help patients with neck pain. The collar can be soft or made from firmer plastazote – this is a very light material.

It is best to wear a neck collar intermittently so that the muscles in that region do not waste. People with neck pain may also be helped by tying a bandage around the middle of the pillow, to make a supporting butterfly pillow.

Diet

Food high in uric acid such as fish roe, sardines and liver may bring on an acute attack of gout but there is no reason to believe that other 'acid' foods such as fruit are harmful in any form of arthritis.

Keep your weight down

When walking, the load on the lower limbs goes up to five times body weight. This means that if you are 28 pounds overweight you carry 140 pounds extra with every step.

DESIRABLE WEIGHT FOR MEN
(aged 25 and over)

Height without shoes		Body frame Small		Body frame Medium		Body frame Large	
ft	in	st	lb	st	lb	st	lb
5	3	8	9	9	7	10	4
5	4	9	0	9	10	10	8
5	5	9	3	9	13	10	12
5	6	9	7	10	3	11	2
5	7	9	11	10	7	11	7
5	8	10	1	10	12	11	12
5	9	10	5	11	2	12	1
5	10	10	10	11	6	12	6
5	11	11	0	11	11	12	11
6	0	11	5	12	2	13	2
6	1	11	8	12	7	13	7
6	2	11	13	12	12	13	12

Weight reduction will benefit your symptoms if you are obese. If you feel that you need help and advice over losing weight, ask your GP to refer you to a dietician. Our chart below will give you an idea of whether you are in the accepted weight range for your height.

Older patients with osteoarthritis may coincidentally have diverticulitis, and those with muscular rheumatism often have irritable bowel syndrome. High fibre diets will benefit these conditions. So try to increase your intake of high fibre foods by eating wholemeal bread, pasta, brown rice, pulses, cereal, fruit and vegetables.

Alcohol (especially heavy red wines) precipitates gout and some other patients with rheumatism find their pains are aggravated by this; otherwise there is no link between drinking and arthritis. Everyone should, however, keep within the guidelines of the Royal College of Physicians of London, which state that the maximum number of units a week for men should be 21 and 14 units for women. A unit is half a pint of beer, a small measure of spirits.

Rheumatoid arthritis

If you have this condition, you're likely to be bombarded with advice about special diets that are supposed to help. You need to be very

DESIRABLE WEIGHT FOR WOMEN
(aged 25 and over)

Height without shoes		Body frame Small		Body frame Medium		Body frame Large	
ft	in	st	lb	st	lb	st	lb
4	11	7	3	7	12	8	10
5	0	7	6	8	1	8	13
5	1	7	9	8	4	9	2
5	2	7	12	8	7	9	5
5	3	8	1	8	10	9	8
5	4	8	4	9	0	9	12
5	5	8	7	9	4	10	2
5	6	8	11	9	9	10	6
5	7	9	0	9	13	10	10
5	8	9	5	10	3	11	0
5	9	9	9	10	7	11	4
5	10	10	0	10	11	11	9

wary of such advice, and discuss any planned change in your diet with your doctor first. In particular, it's worth noting that citrus fruit is not bad for you. It is not 'acid', as is often claimed, and is an important source of vitamin C. Conversely, cod liver oil does not lubricate your joints. It is broken down in the gut long before it ever reaches your joints, and it is likely to make you put on weight. Some people find that certain foods aggravate their symptoms – in which case, it makes sense to avoid them. I advise patients to follow a high fibre diet, restricting, but not excluding, dairy products.

A few of my patients with rheumatism are sensitive to dairy products; but they are only a small group. It is important that everyone should have sufficient vitamins but there is no evidence that supplementary vitamins help to alleviate arthritis. The multiplicity of diets claiming to cure arthritis casts doubt on the value of any. By all means try one, provided it is not deficient in an important constituent, but do not expect too much by way of benefit, and just be grateful if it works.

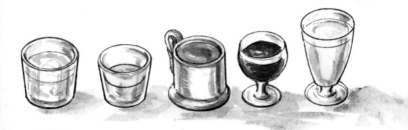

Drugs

W e have few drug cures for arthritis.

An infected joint must be treated in hospital with an antibiotic but the doctor will need to sample the fluid in the joint before selecting an appropriate one.

Acute gout can be controlled rapidly by non-steroidal anti-inflammatory drugs and colchicine. The last is a time-honoured remedy that tends to have side-effects of sickness and diarrhoea – so the patient is made to 'run before he can walk'!

The excess uric acid in the kidneys can be eliminated in the urine by the drugs probenecid or sulphinpyrazone, or by allopurinol which blocks its formation.

These treatments are lifelong and they are only used if acute attacks are frequent, if uric acid deposits are evident, or if the blood concentration of uric acid is persistently very high.

Relieving pain

Pain is the main symptom of most arthritic conditions, and pain-relieving medicines (analgesics) such as paracetamol, aspirin, co-proxamol and ibuprofen may suffice to control this. Locally applied linaments and ointments may also help. If inflammation occurs, drugs are given that relieve pain by acting on this. They are called non-steroidal anti-inflammatory drugs (NSAIDs). Drugs may upset the stomach, particularly in women over 60, and so elderly women should always try analgesics first. If you suffer from asthma you need to be careful in taking NSAIDs because they may aggravate your breathing problems.

Slow-acting anti-rheumatoid drugs

A minority of patients with rheumatoid arthritis need drugs with a more fundamental action on the disease process. They are slow-acting, taking eight to twelve weeks to achieve an effect. They are not used as the first line of treatment and they may modify the course of the disease. These drugs are, therefore, variously called slow-acting anti-rheumatoid drugs, second-line agents or disease modifying drugs.

Examples are sulphasalazine, hydroxychloroquine, gold and d-penicillamine, and all may have side-effects that require watching.

Sulphasalazine causes indigestion in a third of patients; hydroxychloroquine (in large doses) may deposit in the eye if taken for long periods; and gold and d-penicillamine may cause rashes, affect the kidneys, produce protein in the urine, and affect the blood.

Methotrexate is given once a week. At much higher doses it is used as an anti-cancer drug. It is particularly popular in the treatment of rheumatoid arthritis in the USA, and is becoming more so in the UK. Sometimes it causes indigestion, and the state of the blood has to be monitored. It acts more quickly than the other second-line drugs, and if they are withdrawn the arthritis may flare up again.

A sample of the patient's urine has to be checked regularly for protein, therefore, and a blood test has to be taken at regular intervals. The drugs are used when X-rays show joint damage is developing or if the clinical picture or blood test shows that the disease is continuously active for several months.

These drugs are usually safe as long as precautions are taken, but you will need to discuss with your doctor the monitoring of their side-effects.

Steroids

Cortisone-like drugs (steroids) are life-saving in certain rheumatic diseases (such as some forms of systemic lupus erythematosus and polyarteritis nodosa) and in others they may stop the patient going blind (as in temporal arthritis).

Recent work has shown that in small doses they may slow down the course of the disease.

They are used in rheumatoid arthritis if the disease is inexorably progressive or for socio-economic reasons. The breadwinner of the family may have been off work a long time, for instance, or the busy over-worked housewife and mother may be unable to cope.

Unfortunately they have side-effects such as rounding of the face, bruising of the arms and legs, and thinning of the bones, and the dosage must, therefore, be brought as low as possible. Steroids may also aggravate an existing ulcer or produce indigestion.

Under no circumstances should they be stopped suddenly and in the case of surgery or an accident, the dose may need to be increased.

IMMUNOSUPPRESSORS

When severe disorders do not respond to other measures drugs which suppress the immune system may be required. They must be given under close medical supervision.

Every patient on steroids should carry a card, stating the drug and the dose they are receiving. The anti-inflammatory effect of steroids is best when they are placed at the site of inflammation by injection. They will often cure a tennis elbow, or alleviate the pain of periarthritis of the shoulder. If one or two joints only are inflamed they will cause these to settle when injected into the cavity. They are seldom used in osteoarthritis, unless there is considerable inflammation in the joint or a local patch of inflammation around the joint margin, when an injection into the site may be given. An injection into the base of the thumbs can be helpful if these are affected. The treatment should not be given too often in case the injection damages the joint; and it is best to rest the joint for 48 hours after an injection.

Supplementary drugs

Additional drugs may be necessary to treat other aspects of the disease such as iron for anaemia, antidepressive drugs and calcium in an endeavour to stem bone loss. Drugs which cause the muscles to relax are also used.

New developments

There is a lot of research being done by the pharmaceutical industry and university researchers on new drugs designed to benefit patients with arthritis. One approach has been to identify those substances which play a part in the chemical cascade that produces inflammation. Drugs are being developed to block these substances.

Researchers are also using techniques developed in recent years, such as monoclonal antibodies, but they are still in the experimental stage. The drugs often have to be given into the vein and the benefit only lasts for a few weeks. They are, nevertheless, exciting developments which are likely to pave the way for a whole new generation of helpful – possibly even curative – drugs.

Surgery

Tendons repaired

Ruptured tendons may be repaired and lumps (nodules) in patients with arthritis can be removed, but unfortunately these often recur.

Synovectomy

The diseased lining of a joint, such as the knee, may be removed if it has been chronically inflamed for several months and if the joint itself is not damaged. This operation is known as synovectomy. Should this be the major joint affected, that would be an added reason for this operation. The pain of two-thirds of the patients is relieved for several years by this procedure but it is a major operation and the joint takes some time to regain its former movement.

Osteotomy

This is when the bone is cut to realign the joint. It is sometimes done at the knee when it has become misshapen (causing bow legs or knock knees) or at the hip in younger patients. About two-thirds of the patients do well for several years with this procedure. The joint itself is not entered, and more elaborate surgery can be done later if needed.

Arthrodesis

This is the stiffening of a joint. A frail rheumatoid thumb can be brought back to valuable function in this way and a rheumatoid wrist may benefit from stiffing. Often a little very painful movement is worse than a painless wrist stiffened in a slightly extended position. Occasionally it is done for a knee, when that is the only joint affected and it is giving great pain. If infection has occurred previously, a surgeon would prefer to stiffen a joint rather than replace it.

Arthroplasty

This is the replacement of a joint.

Normal hip joint

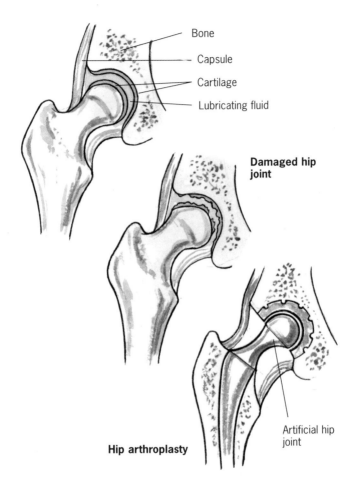

Bone

Capsule

Cartilage

Lubricating fluid

Damaged hip joint

Hip arthroplasty

Artificial hip joint

Diagram comparing a normal hip joint, a damaged hip joint, and a hip joint replacement (arthroplasty)

The simplest form is excision arthroplasty in which the end of the bone is removed and fibrous tissue grows between the two surfaces. This is commonly done at the ball of the feet for severe rheumatoid arthritis. It is called a Fowler's operation and results are usually good. The end of the smaller bone at the wrist may be removed when it is roughened and has been rubbing up against nearby tendons and when it is causing pain in the wrist. Excision arthroplasty is occasionally done at the hip, with the removal of the head of the thigh bone or femur (a Girdlestone operation) when a rheumatoid patient is already confined to a wheelchair, has a very painful hip, and other affected joints which would stop him or her walking with an artificial hip.

JOINT REPLACEMENT

By arthroplasty, we usually mean replacement of one or both joint surfaces with artificial material. The biggest single advance in the treatment of arthritis this century has been the development of adequate hip replacement (prosthesis) and the lives of thousands of patients with osteoarthritis and rheumatoid arthritis of the hip have been transformed by this operation. Two features have helped in its success. The first is the development of materials to make a low friction joint. Early arthroplasties used metal rubbing on metal. Because the joint is bathed in body

Knee replacement

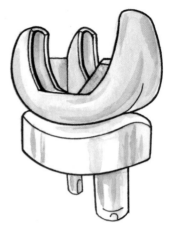

Replacement of the knee joint now rivals hip replacement as a treatment for arthritis. Tough plastic materials are used to provide new surfaces for the bones making the upper and lower parts of the joint

fluids which contain chemicals, both joint surfaces had to be made of the same metal, otherwise an electrolytic cell would be produced resulting in corrosion. The same metals rubbing together have poor 'slidability' (a high coefficient of friction) so that occasionally these joints would stick. They also tended to loosen more rapidly than later arthroplasties.

Metal and plastic

Most hip arthroplasties today use a metal component in the thigh bone, which fits in a plastic socket in the pelvis. This combination has a low coefficient of friction and the modern plastics wear well. These designs are based on the pioneer work in Whittington Hospital by the late Professor Sir John Charnley.

Plastic cement

A second important feature is that the components are locked into position by plastic cement. This means that the patient can be mobilised quickly. New prostheses made of ceramics are being used. Because they wear less quickly, they are sometimes used in young people requiring joint replacement.

However some prostheses are coated to stimulate the bone to grow into it. This avoids more foreign material in the body and anchors the prosthesis solidly. However, recovery takes longer and the prosthesis may be difficult to remove if need be.

A major procedure

Replacing a hip is a major procedure not to be undertaken lightly. The orthopaedic surgeon will want to know if your general health is good and in particular whether your heart and lungs are in good working order. If you are a smoker or are overweight, that may deter him. He will want to know whether the other joints of your legs are in sufficiently good condition for you to benefit from surgery to the hip.

Above all, he will want to be sure your arthritis is sufficiently severe to warrant hip arthroplasty. He will be guided in the main by the amount of pain you experience. If this is severe, and if it disturbs your sleep, he will regard that as a major indication.

WAITING LISTS

If you have been accepted for hip arthroplasty, often after discussion between a rheumatologist and an orthopaedic surgeon, your name will be put on the waiting list and when a bed becomes available you will be notified.

However, you may have to wait between three and eighteen months, depending on the size of the waiting lists in your district.

Interestingly, this pain may be felt mainly at the knee, although that joint may be normal (this is called referred pain). The surgeon will want to be sure that the pain is not coming from your back, because wear and tear in the spine can sometimes produce pain in the hip region. Another factor he will take into account is how much the hip limits your movements. If your complaint is mainly of limited movement with little pain, he will probably wish to defer the operation and monitor your progress.

Sometimes, however, hip movement may be so limited that it interferes with toilet function and sexual activity. That will be taken into account.

Age – an important consideration

Surgeons prefer to operate on patients aged 55 or over, but every year, more and more younger people are having successful hip replacement operations. Newer techniques don't use cement, but instead require new bone to grow into the prosthesis to keep it in the correct position. Several studies have given encouraging early results, but it will be a while before we can assess how long they last.

The success rate, particularly in relieving pain, is high (ninety per cent or more) but nevertheless complications do occur. Every operation has its risks and hip arthroplasty is no exception. Sometimes, despite strict precautions, infection occurs and this is why surgeons are reluctant to operate on anyone with infection of the urinary tract or the chest or a leg ulcer.

Infection may also happen at a later stage (sometimes many months after the operation). We do not know whether a pocket of infection is left at operation or whether (more likely) a germ from the bloodstream lodges in the joint. The infection may clear with antibiotics but sometimes it necessitates the removal of the prosthesis. The patient is then left with an excision arthroplasty, which will be pain-free, but the joint will be much less stable. If the femoral component loosens after some years it may have to be removed but another can be put in its place. Surgeons are reluctant to replace an infected prosthesis because these often become infected again.

Occasionally the prosthesis dislocates but this is usually rectified easily. Again, on rare occasions, bone may grow around the prosthesis giving an unsatisfactory result and the operation may have to be redone.

The operation

On admission to hospital preliminary checks will be done, and usually the hip will be replaced within two or three days. Different surgeons have different policies about the programme of care after the operation. Many like their patients to lie flat in bed for a few days with their legs separated by a pillow. Within a week you will be out of bed and walking with the help of nurses or physiotherapists; within two weeks you will probably be home: and after three months you will be returning to normal. The pain will have gone and your hip will have a much better range of movement, although it may not regain full motion. You should notify your doctor if you experience unusual hip or chest pain, if you notice persistent swelling of the legs, if you develop a temperature, or if you notice any oozing from the site of your wound.

Convalescence

Immediately after the operation do not sit or squat, or bend your legs up in bed. The doctor will tell you when it is safe to sit out using a high chair and when to lie on your side at night. In the first three months at home avoid lying on the operated side. Sit on a high firm chair with arm rests, keep your knees and feet apart, and sit for short periods of not more than 30 minutes, getting up periodically to walk round.

Avoid leaning forward more than 90 degrees and don't cross your legs. Use your feet to turn and take short frequent walks. If you go for a long walk, use a stick on the unoperated side. Go up stairs with your unoperated leg first, then the operated leg, then your stick. Reverse the procedure going down stairs, putting your stick first, then the operated leg, and then the unoperated leg. It is better to use a shower rather than a bath and avoid slippery surfaces. Most patients undergoing this surgery are delighted with the results. Sexual activity can be resumed after six to eight weeks and the most sensible position is lying on your back.

Knee surgery

Great advances have been made in this type of surgery, and diagnosis has been greatly improved by the development of an instrument called the arthroscope. This is a small, telescope-like gadget which is inserted through a small incision and allows the doctor to examine the knee internally and see whether the menisci have been torn, whether the synovial lining is inflamed, whether the cartilage covering the bone is damaged or whether loose fragments of bone or cartilage are present. The arthroscope has been refined so that small pieces of tissue can be obtained for microscopic examination (biopsy). Operations can also be performed through it, so that in some cases a damaged meniscus can be removed (menisectomy) without recourse to opening up the joint.

Osteoarthritis of the knee is a major problem, and patients normally complain first of pain and stiffness in their knees. Sometimes, however, the main symptom is locking of the knee, when the joint becomes stuck in a particular position and can only be loosened by a sudden movement. The cause may be either the presence of loose fragments of bone which have broken off inside the joint, or a degeneration of the cartilage in the knee, which may be torn, possibly as a result of an injury. You'll usually be sent for an

ARTHROPLASTY OF THE KNEE

Many different types of knee arthroplasty have been developed. They usually cover the lower end of the femur with a metal shell, which articulates on a plastic disc covering the top of the shin bone (tibia). Because the knee is nearer the surface than the hip and is much more complex, it poses greater problems in terms of wound healing, infection, and recovery of the full range of movement. Nevertheless, the results of knee replacement operations have improved greatly in recent years, and many thousands of patients have benefited. Once again, pain is the main reason for doing the operation.

X-ray, to see whether there are any fragments in the joint, followed by an arthroscopy. This involves keyhole surgery during which the surgeon looks into the joint and carries out the appropriate treatment. The possibilities are:

- Loose fragments can be removed
- A torn cartilage can be removed
- Any cartilage lying in the joint which appears to be causing a mechanical problem can be trimmed or where the cartilage is worn down nearly to the bone, it can be scraped away to help with pain relief
- The joint can be washed out.

Arthroscopy solves the problem of locking; following a joint washout, fifty per cent of people will have their symptoms relieved which delays the need for further surgery.

Sometimes, only one side of the knee is noticeably affected when you have osteoarthritis. In patients aged below 55, surgeons will often carry out an osteotomy – an operation to realign the knee and so relieve pain, although this does deal with the underlying problem which is responsible for the symptoms. The advantage is that it can delay the need for joint replacement for several years. Similarly, if only one side of the knee is affected, some surgeons will perform what is called an unicondylar knee replacement, which only replaces one half of the knee joint, but does relieve the symptoms.

The knee has two strong internal ligaments which cross (hence the name cruciate) and help to stabilise the knee. A ligament may be ruptured in an accident or in the sort of sporting injury sustained by Paul Gascoigne while playing for Spurs in the Cup Final. Not only does the rupture cause intense pain and instability of the joint, but it may also lead to osteoarthritis. These ligaments can be repaired, either by using tissue from another part of the body or by an artificial ligament which stimulates the growth of the natural ligament. Gascoigne was treated by the first method and Graham Bell, the British Olympic skier, by the second.

The replacement of knees damaged by rheumatoid arthritis or osteoarthritis (knee arthroplasty) has developed considerably in recent years. The results are as good as those from hip replacement operations, and figures from work in North Yorkshire suggest that there will be a great demand from patients to have this treatment on the NHS. Finally, though, a cautionary note: if a hip replacement goes wrong, as inevitably a few will, the situation can be easily salvaged. If a knee replacement goes wrong, that poses a very real problem, and in very rare cases, may even require amputation. Unfortunately, you may be one of those people for whom a knee replacement operation is not suitable. This is usually because the knee is too seriously damaged or the joint is too deformed. In this situation, the only way to relieve pain is to fuse the joint by a process called arthrodesis. This will leave you with a stiff leg because you can no longer move your knee, but at least you will be free of pain in the joint.

As in the hip, arthroplasty is usually the best available treatment for a painful knee, especially when it is causing significant disability. Over recent years, advances in the design of knee replacement joints have raised the long-term success rate for this form of surgery so that it is now comparable to hip replacement. As with hip operations, there is always the possibility of infection, so the same precautions have to be taken.

Usually, plastic cement is used to hold the components of the new joint in place, although new techniques have been developed which make this unnecessary. This is especially useful for younger patients, as it makes it easier to replace the joint if it eventually wears out. The problem rarely arises with older people as the joint components will normally last for as long as they are needed.

The operation

Once you're in hospital, you will spend two or three days undergoing checks before you have the operation. Afterwards, your knee will be put into a machine which bends it for you. You'll probably find it painful at first, but this should wear off after a few days as you begin to feel the benefit. The aim is to get your knee to bend at right angles before you leave hospital. At first, your joint will be protected by a brace, but once you can lift your leg without bending the knee, you'll be allowed to walk without the brace. Your stitches will normally come out after 12 days, and you'll be given the same advice about caring for the scars as someone who's had a hip replacement (see page 39).

Getting over it

Once again, the situation is much the same as it is for people convalescing after a hip replacement. You can normally travel by car as a passenger almost immediately, but you'll be advised not to drive yourself for three months or so.

Plastic knuckles

Plastic knuckles have been developed which do not give a greater range of movement to the fingers but abolish pain. If the fingers are very deformed arthroplasties will improve the appearance – a factor that may be important to many people. Sometimes the prosthesis breaks and has to be replaced but this is not difficult.

Shoulders, elbows and ankles

Arthroplasties for the shoulder, elbow and ankle have been developed but pose greater problems. After shoulder replacement the patient may be unable to move the artificial joint through the full range of movement, probably due to damage which has already occurred to the surrounding muscles and tendons. For this reason a shoulder prosthesis will move better if it is done for an injury than if it is done for arthritis.

General principles of joint protection

Living with arthritis

Making changes in the way you live and around the home is not 'giving in to arthritis', it is simply good sense. There are many ways in which you can put less strain on your joints and reduce the amount of pain you get. Often, a few changes will enable you to lead a fuller life.

Identify any triggering factors and avoid aggravating them

Patients with neck and shoulder girdle pain should avoid carrying heavy shopping or baggage or lifting heavy things such as furniture or heavy equipment.

Remember that vigorous games of tennis or badminton are highly likely to provoke a recurrence of tennis elbow. Walking over fell country, rough ground, or cobbled streets and even climbing stairs will aggravate osteoarthritis of the knees or hips. If you wish to do these kind of activities you must decide whether the gains are worth the possible pain.

Use the strongest and largest joint possible to do a task

Remember that the palm or forearm can often be used instead of arthritic fingers. Ladies, for instance, can carry their handbag on a forearm or use a shoulder bag to avoid clutching it in an arthritic hand.

To lift heavy objects from the floor, bend your knees instead of your back!

Distribute a load over several joints

If your arms, for example, have arthritis, use both to push and pull and use both hands to hold or carry things.

Use good body mechanics

Each joint should be used in its most stable and functional position when

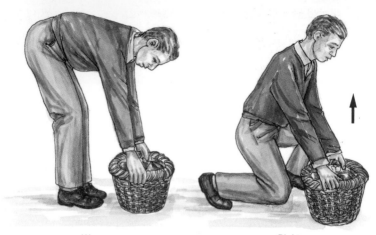

Wrong

Right

possible. The hand is most effective, for example, when the wrist is bent slightly backwards.

A splint may be needed to keep a joint in the functional position. A Futura wrist splint, for instance, can actually enable a patient with painful wrists to work.

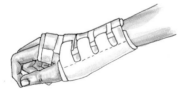

Futura wrist splint

Don't avoid things that assist the joints

A stick should not be regarded as a badge of crippledom. It more than

halves the load on a damaged leg joint.

Avoid a chair that sags. A chair should be easy to rise from and that

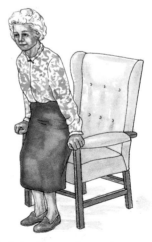

A chair with arms is easy to rise from

REDUCE THE EFFORT REQUIRED TO DO A JOB IN THE KITCHEN

- Wide handles for cutlery make gripping easier. Specially designed cutlery is available, but often padding around the handles of standard implements is all that is needed.

- Have lever arm taps, or a tap turner attached to the normal fitting.

- Stop bowls and plates sliding by putting them on a damp cloth, or fitting suction pads.

- Buy as much electrical equipment as you can afford, such as can openers, food mixers and processors, knives and scissors which only require squeezing.

- Reduce the distance you need to go to obtain materials and minimise bending. When you replace your refrigerator, for instance, consider a table top model and have cupboards easily accessible.

- Washing machines and microwave ovens take the drudgery out of the healthy person's life and they ease the burden of the arthritic person's lot, too. Tools for living help everyone.

- Drop a few hints to your devoted children about what mother or father would appreciate for Christmas.

requires a high seat (if necessary put blocks under the legs). Arms on a chair can also reduce the load on your legs considerably when rising.

Modified shoes may help painful feet. If the balls of the feet hurt, bars on the outside of the soles or metatarsal insoles will help and made-to-measure shoes are a great boon to those with greater foot deformity. Surgical shoes are no longer the unsightly black boots of olden days. Stylish shoes and boots are now available and if you need these, two pairs are provided by the NHS and an additional pair each year afterwards.

A car with power steering and automatic gears will help a patient with arthritis in the arm joints. If neck

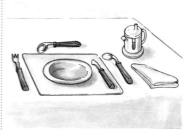

movement is limited, a panorama rear view mirror gives good vision. A 'Super Scope Mirror' can be purchased cheaply from the National Ankylosing Spondylitis Society (the address is on page 53). The mirror can be returned if it is not suitable for the vehicle.

Around the house

Your house or flat may be inconvenient for someone with arthritis, but you should think very carefully before considering moving to a bungalow or modern building. Moving is always expensive, especially in an economic recession and is often upsetting, especially for elderly people. You are familiar with your own neighbours, shopkeepers, postman and milkman and it is not easy to adjust to a new neighbourhood. Some modifications to settle into your current home may be a cheaper and better solution that will enable you to continue living there.

Many people with arthritis find that getting up and down stairs is exhausting and painful. Accidents

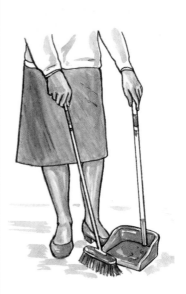

are common on steep stairs, especially if the lighting is poor.

● Make sure the stair carpet is firmly fixed with no holes in it and fit a strong lightbulb and use it.

● You may need a rail on both sides if you are unsteady.

● If you find the stairs are exhausting or painful, one solution,

DISABLED LIVING CENTRE

If you have a Disabled Living Centre in your town, visit it. There is a great variety of appliances available for inspection and trial and trained staff will help and advise. You cannot purchase the aids there, but the centre shows what is available. You must make an appointment by telephone or by letter. Look in Yellow Pages.

cheaper than moving house or even fitting a downstairs toilet, is to install an electric stair lift.

Modern lifts take up very little space and can be fitted to virtually any staircase, straight or curved. The lift rail is fixed to the stairs, not the wall, and requires no structural alterations. Fitting a lift takes only a few hours.

Many other minor modifications can be made which will make your daily tasks much easier and often safer.

● Have electric sockets raised to an accessible height and, where possible, adapt switches to make them easy to use.

● Use long-handled dustpans and brushes; and replace stiff door knobs with lever handles.

● Avoid small mats or rugs, folds in the carpet, and tears in the lino.

● Buy a 'helping hand' (a long handle with a magnet on the end), or lazy tongs which extend to the floor and will pick up objects as small as a pencil.

● Install a push button telephone and an entry phone; this saves effort and improves security.

In the bathroom

A bath board may help you to get into the bath and a bath seat will help if you cannot get down in one movement. Put non-slip material on

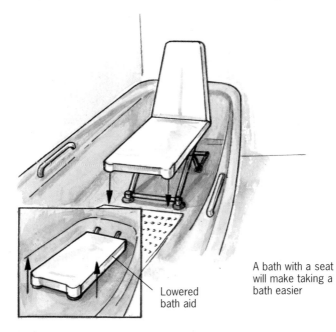

Lowered bath aid

A bath with a seat will make taking a bath easier

the bottom of the bath and have a rail attached to the wall to help you get out. A shower can be much easier to use than a bath. A raised toilet seat is a great help if movement in your hips or knees is limited and a rail alongside will help you rise.

One occupational therapy student wrote in her exam paper: 'Every rheumatic patient is helped by a bar in the toilet.' I think she meant a rail!

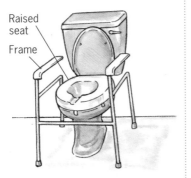

Raised seat

Frame

A raised toilet seat with armrests is a great help

In the garden

Use long-handled tools, don't be tempted into heavy digging, and do remember it is often better to kneel on a mat to do a job than doing it standing up.

At work

Think how you can modify your work pattern to minimise stress on the joints, and discuss any suggestions

IN THE BEDROOM

- Raise the bed to the level most easy for you to get in and out.
- Use a duvet rather than heavy blankets to keep warm at night.
- If you are having disturbed nights then two single beds pushed together may be more satisfactory than one double bed. Or a double bed with a slatted wooden base may be the answer. Sleeping separately may help the well partner, but the ill person may feel isolated and unhappy.
- Clothing can be made to fasten at the front rather than the back and Velcro makes a better fastening than buckles, tight buttons, or press studs.
- A long-handled stocking aid and shoe horn help deal with socks and shoes.
- Elastic shoe-laces overcome the need to tie knots.

with the boss. (Often it improves efficiency.)

One factory I visited required my patient to hit a button with his wrist hundreds of times daily to open a small gate. We modified the apparatus so that he could knock a lever with his forearm instead. This

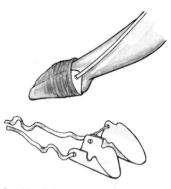

Stocking helper

speeded up production to the delight of the management and the worker. An occupational therapist may also arrange to visit a place of work to suggest modification to your employer.

Avoid prolonged periods in one position

Patients with any type of arthritis will stiffen up if they stay in one position for a long time. Never sit for longer than one hour without getting up and just walking around the room. This will help loosen up stiffening joints.

Avoid positions and activities leading to possible joint deformity

Never put a pillow under your knees at night; permanently bent knees may result. If the knees have active arthritis, rest splints from the occupational therapist may well keep them in a good position at night. Similarly, splints for the wrists and the hands help to prevent deformity.

Organise your work and eliminate needless tasks

Happy is the housewife whose husband is a handy man. He can modify the kitchen to minimise her efforts. Organise work efficiently and balance it with rest. If dusting tires you out, find someone else to do it or remove some of your ornaments.

If ironing exhausts you forget about the tea towels and sheets. Let dishes drip dry and don't worry if the house has a 'lived-in' appearance; it is more welcoming that way.

Remember chiropody

In a survey of 100 patients with arthritis I found that half required chiropody. Taking care of the feet can make life so much more comfortable, so do visit the chiropodist. Be careful about the removal of corns under the ball of the foot, however, as they are the body's protection for fallen joints.

Evaluate 'unorthodox' remedies carefully before using them

Homeopathy is a system of medicine founded by Samuel Hahnemann of Leipzig in about 1876. It treats diseases by the addition of minute doses of drugs which would produce similar symptoms in a healthy person to those caused by the disease. Some doctors have claimed good results from this approach and use it in combination with conventional treatment.

Acupuncture has helped a few of my patients, but not many. Copper bracelets make pleasant ornaments, and will do you no harm. Spiritual healing has been in the news. No sensible person ignores the spiritual dimension in their life and certainly, inner bitterness and resentment can aggravate your physical condition. Whether spiritual healing and yoga, which are advocated as adjuncts to orthodox medicine, are helpful, however, has yet to be proved. The global claims of faith healers who declare that all illness can be cured provided that you have sufficient faith is false to the *Bible* and to experience. They are particularly dangerous if they advocate the sudden stopping of all medicine as the demonstration of your faith.

When confronted by 'fringe medicine', note who makes the claims: ask are they supported by any evidence other than testimonials; and enquire how much money the practitioner will make out of it. To raise the hopes of someone with a chronic illness unjustifiably is cruel.

The future

For most forms of arthritis there is a positive outlook and it is a great relief to sufferers to realise that even in their 90s they are unlikely to be in a wheelchair. This is especially true for sufferers from generalised osteoarthritis. Many women consult me with painful lumps on their fingers, thinking they have rheumatoid arthritis. I explain that the sequence of events is that the pain will subside, leaving them with lumps which may impair their glamour but not their function. They all avow that they are not concerned about their glamour, which is not true, but their relief is such that they believe it at that moment. Others think that because their joints crack or creak, they too are bound for the wheelchair. They are not: this does not indicate developing arthritis.

Agonising conditions like gout can be cured

The considerable pain of a condition like periarthritis of the shoulder can be alleviated quickly, although it may take two or three years for the full range of joint movement to be restored, and eighty-five per cent of patients with ankylosing spondylitis never have a day off work.

Rheumatoid arthritis can be controlled

Nor is rheumatoid arthritis necessarily a crippling disorder. In a survey we did in Wensleydale, many patients had rheumatoid arthritis of such mild degree that they had not even consulted their general practitioner, let alone a specialist. A study in Edinburgh of patients with disease sufficiently severe for them to be admitted to hospital, showed that after ten years, four out of every ten were either free from symptoms or had only minor troubles. Only relatively few develop deformities and even then deformity and incapacity are not the same. Some of the most beautiful embroidery I possess was done by rheumatoid patients whose hands were gnarled and distorted by arthritis. Much can be done to control this disease and prevent deformities.

FINAL WORD

Although much of this book has concentrated on severe disease, it should be emphasised that most forms of arthritis are not crippling. For all patients, the adequate treatment is a combined venture between you and your doctor. Several promising lines of research are being pursued by university departments of rheumatology and the pharmaceutical industry to produce treatments which will ameliorate the suffering caused by these diseases and provide a cure.

Useful information

Arthritis Care
18 Stephenson Way
London NW1 2HD
Helpline: 0808 8004050 (12am–4pm
Mon–Fri)
Tel: 020 7916 1500
Fax: 020 7916 1505
Email: arthritis-care@virgin.net
Website: www.arthritiscare.org

Provides information, advice and practical aid to people with arthritis. Has branches throughout the country and publishes a regular paper *Arthritis News* for its members.

Arthritis Research Campaign
Copeman House, St Mary's Court
Chesterfield S41 7TD
Tel: 01246 558033
Fax: 01246 558007
Email: info@arc.org.uk
Website: www.arc.org.uk

Finances an extensive programme of research and education and produces over 60 helpful booklets, available from the ARC, your GP or your rheumatologist. Produces a number of videos and publishes a quarterly magazine, *Arthritis Today*, for the general public.

Back Care
16 Elmtree Road
Teddington
Middx TW11 8ST
Tel: 020 8977 5474
Fax: 020 8943 5318
Email: back_pain@compuserve.com
Website: www.backpain.org

Raises funds to support research into the causes and treatment of back pain, and to help alleviate and prevent back pain by teaching people to use their bodies sensibly. Local branches disseminate information and provide neighbourly help to people with back pain.

Disabled Living Foundation
380–384 Harrow Road
London W9 2HU
Helpline: 0870 603 9177 (10am–4pm
Mon–Fri)
Tel: 020 7289 6111
Minicom: 0870 603 9176
Fax: 020 7266 2922
Email: dlfinfo@dlf.org.uk
Website: www.dlf.org.uk

Gives unbiased advice and information on choosing daily living equipment for disability. There are a number of centres around the country. Visits to their equipment display centre can be arranged by appointment.

National Ankylosing Spondylitis Society
PO Box 179, Mayfield
East Sussex TN20 6ZL
Tel: 01435 873527
Fax: 01435 873027
Email: nass@nass.co.uk
Website: www.nass.co.uk

A society for people with ankylosing spondylitis, their families and friends, and doctors and research societies working in the field. Aims include educating patients, professions and the public in the problems of the disease. It has over 100 branches nationwide, providing weekly supervised physiotherapy. Publishes a twice yearly journal for members and a useful guidebook for patients. A cassette tape of physiotherapy exercises and a video (*Fight Back*) about the disease are also available.

Psoriatic Arthropathy Alliance
PO Box 111
St Albans AL2 3JQ
Tel: 01923 672837
Fax: 01923 672837
Email: office@paalliance.org
Website: www.paalliance.org

Provides information and support for those with psoriatic arthropathy. Publishes a quarterly newsletter, information sheets and booklets.

USEFUL LINKS

British Society for Rheumatology
www.rheumatology.org.uk

The Information for Patients section includes publications of interest and links to and contact details of support groups

HealthInFocus (Medicom International Ltd)
www.healthinfocus.co.uk

Aims to provide facts about a disease, how you can expect to be treated, the level of medical care you can expect and the treatments you are likely to receive in the UK.

Index